Diabetic
Cookbook

For a Carefree Life. Quick and Easy
Recipes to Stay Healthy, Boost Energy
and Live Better

Additionally, the information in the following pages is intended only for informational purposes and should thus be thought of as universal. As befitting its nature, it is presented without assurance regarding its prolonged validity or interim quality. Trademarks that are mentioned are done without written consent and can in no way be considered an endorsement from the trademark holder.

Disclaimer

The content, writing, images, photos, descriptions and information contained in this book are for general guidance and are intended for informational purposes only for the readers. The author has narrated his cooking and research experiences in this book by observing and evaluating relevant facts and figures. The author is not a registered dietitian and nutritional information in this book should only be used as a general guideline. Statements in this book have not been evaluated or approved by any regulatory authority.
The author has tried to provide all the information related to the ingredients, foods, and products, however, when certain ingredients get mixed, they may create some kind of cross-reaction which may cause allergy among some people. There may be products that will not be gluten-free and may contain ingredients that may cause a reaction. These products may include but are limited to, eggs, dairy, wheat, nuts, coconut, flour, soy, cocoa, milk, sugar, and other products. These may cause allergic reactions in some people due to cross-contamination from allergen-causing products. The readers and purchasers of this book understand and consent that there may be ingredients in the foods which may contain certain allergens and the readers and purchasers hereby disclaimer the author of this book from all liabilities related to allergic and cross food reactions.

The information provided in this book must not be taken as an alternative to any advice by a doctor, physician, dietitian or health care specialist. The readers should not use the information given in this book for diagnosing an illness or other health-related problems. Furthermore, the readers also should not discontinue professional medical or healthcare advice because of something they have read in this book. The content and information provided in this book do not create any kind of professional relationship between the reader and the author of this book.

This book in no way provides any warranty, express or implied, towards the content of recipes contained in this book. It is the reader's responsibility to determine the value and quality of any recipe or instructions provided for food preparation and to determine the nutritional value if any, and safety of the preparation instructions. Therefore, the author of this book is not responsible for the outcome of any recipe that a reader may try from this book. The readers of this book may not always have the same results due to variations in ingredients, humidity, altitude, cooking temperatures, errors, omissions, or individual cooking abilities.

The images and photos contained in this book may have been used for representational, informative and information purposes and may not be the exact match of the accompanying recipes. These images and photos provide the author's impression of how a particular recipe might look after it has been cooked, made or completed and the images and photos should only be relied upon for the purpose of reference and not actual finished products, recipes or foods.

By purchasing this book, readers hereby acknowledge that they are going to rely on any information provided in the book 'as-is' and must not use this information to form any final conclusion, whether the information is in the form of description, recipe, or ingredient.

Readers agree that they will consult a physician, dietitian or professional healthcare specialist before using and relying on any data, information, or suggestion described in this book.

—

Table of Contents

Living healthy with diabetes

With the complete information included in this cookbook, you will see that the goal is to help you feel in control of your diabetes. The easy-to-follow recipes will help you to live healthy with diabetes.

Eat healthy, live healthy!

Introduction

The word "diabetes" is so scary! To understand the diabetes, it is essential to understand how your body consumes insulin and glucose. Glucose is a form of sugar, and it is the main fuel that the body needs and uses for energy. It is getting ready when the food you eat is broken down during digestion. Moreover, glucose passes through the bloodstream and enters into the cells of the body with the help of insulin. Insulin is a hormone, and it is made in the pancreas. It can be said the insulin is a "key" that opens the cells so that glucose can go inside and provide energy to the body.

Diabetes develops when insulin is completely absent. If diabetes is not diagnosed and treated, different diseases will affect your body, such as blindness, heart, blood vessel disease, stroke, kidney failure, nerve damage, and limb amputation. But, if you will take care of your diabetes and eat the right foods, take your medication regularly, if prescribed, and exercise regularly, you will stay healthy.

My cookbook has a collection of original diabetes recipes for you. These recipes are authentic and healthy for you. In each recipe, easy-to-find ingredients, simple and step-by-step cooking instructions, and additional tips are included. My goal is that you will live healthily and eat healthy with diabetes.

I added four chapters in this cookbook for everyday meals. Such as

- Breakfast recipes
- Lunch recipes
- Dinner recipes
- Dessert recipes

My goal with this cookbook is to have an easier time preparing healthy meals for your family and friends.

I have included important information that needs you to understand and control diabetes with two healthy meal plans for your good health.

So, let's begin!

Tips for living healthy with diabetes:

- Do not overeat
- Do not skip meal
- Choose healthy foods that are high in nutrients and low in calories
- Do exercise regularly

Avoid foods:

There are many foods and beverages that should avoid in diabetes type 2. There are followings:

Salty or fried foods	High fat dairy products	Shellfish	Food high is saturated fat or trans fat
White rice or pasta	Bake products such as white bread and bagels	Processed meats	Processed snacks
Sweet fruits – for example fruit juices	Shortening and margarine	Organ meats such as, beef or liver	

Eat Foods:

Tuna	Sweet potatoes	Halibut	Almonds, pecans, and walnuts
Cod	Legumes such as beans	Flaxseeds	
Non starchy vegetables	Quinoa or oats	Mackerel	
Whole fruits	Sardines	Olive oil, canola oil, and peanut oil	

Healthy ingredients for diabetes

Vegetables:
One cup raw or half cup

Dandelion green	Beet greens
Mustard green	Collard greens

Non-starchy vegetables:
High cup cooked or one cup raw:

Onion	Bell pepper	Mushrooms
Tomato	Celery	Garlic
Zucchini	Carrot	
Fennel	Okra	

Root or starchy vegetable:

Cassava flour - 1/2 cup, cooked	Pumpkin – 1 cup, cooked	Sweet potatoes – ½ cup, cooked
Potato – ½ cup, cooked	Sweet peas – ½ cup, cooked	

Fruit:

Peach	Lime	Orange
Pineapple	Lemon	Apple
Strawberries	Banana	

Grain:

Red rice	Quinoa	Teff – ½ cup, cooked
Cornmeal	Brown rice	

Legume and beans:

Black beans	Lima beans	Pinto beans
Black-eyed peas	Kidney beans	
Butter beans	Chickpeas flour	

Diary:

Butternut	Plain yogurt	Fat-free milk

Nuts:

Almond flour	Peanuts

Healthy fats:

Extra-virgin olive oil	Sunflower seed oil	Coconut milk

About recipes:

These diabetes recipes are tasty and healthy. You can choose a recipe for an everyday meal – breakfast, lunch, dinner, and dessert. You can prepare these meals easily for your family because all recipes are simple to prepare.

After eating these meals, you will comment:

- I will enjoy this meal!
- I feel healthy and active now!

Breakfast recipes

Breakfast Avocado-Egg Toast

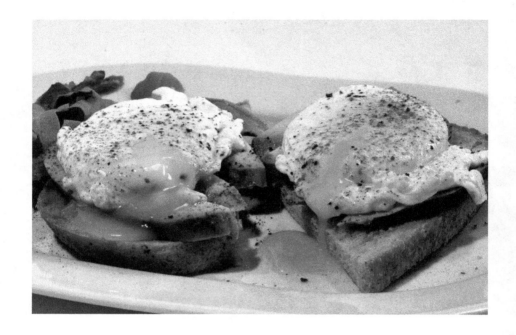

Preparation time: 5 minutes
Serving: 1

Ingredients:

- Avocado – ¼
- Ground pepper – ¼ tsp
- Garlic powder – 1/8 tsp
- Whole-wheat bread – 1 slice, toasted
- Egg – one, fried
- Sriracha – one tsp, optional
- Scallion – one tbsp, sliced, optional

Instructions:

- Mix the garlic powder, pepper, and avocado into the bowl. Mash it.
- Top toast with the fried egg and avocado mixture.
- Top with scallions and sriracha.
- Serve!

Additional Tip:

- Garnish with sliced avocado.

Breakfast Spinach and Egg Scramble

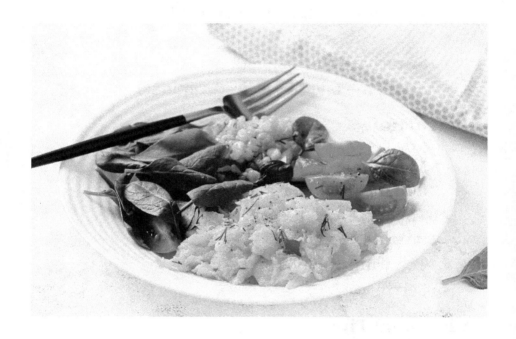

Preparation time: 10 minutes
Serving: 1

Ingredients:

- Canola oil – one tsp
- Baby spinach – 1 ½ cup
- Eggs – two, beaten
- Pinch of kosher salt
- Pinch of ground pepper
- Whole-grain bread – one slice, toasted
- Fresh raspberries – half cup

Instructions:

- Add oil into the skillet and heat over medium-high flame.
- Then, add spinach and cook for one to two minutes.
- Transfer the spinach to the medium plate.
- Clean the pan and add eggs and cook over medium flame. Cook for one to two minutes until set. Add in pepper, salt, and spinach.

Additional Tip:

- Serve with toasted raspberries.

Pistachio and Peach Toast

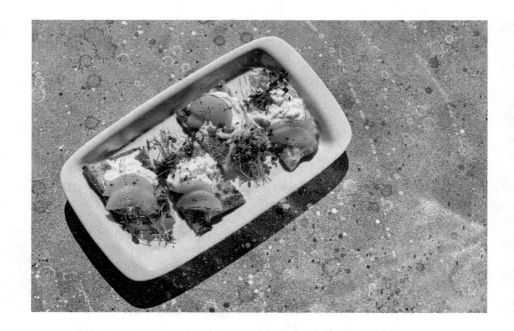

Preparation time: 5 minutes
Serving: 1

Ingredients:

- Part-skim ricotta cheese – one tbsp
- Honey – one tsp
- Cinnamon – 1/8 tsp
- Whole-wheat bread – one slice, toasted
- Peach – half, sliced
- Pistachios – one tbsp, chopped

Instructions:

- Mix the cinnamon, half tsp honey, and ricotta into the bowl.
- Scatter ricotta mixture over the toast.
- Top with pistachios and peaches.
- Drizzle with half tsp honey.
- Serve!

Additional Tip:

- Sprinkle with pistachios.

Peanut Butter and chia Berry Jam muffin

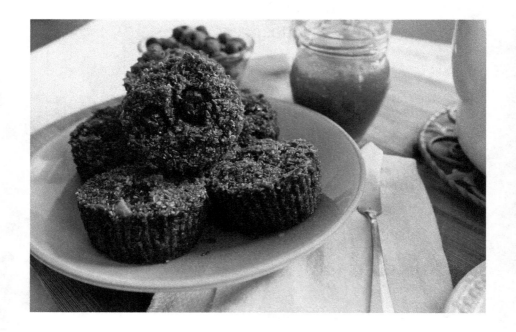

Preparation time: 10 minutes
Serving: 1

Ingredients:

- Unsweetened mixed frozen berries – half cup
- Chia seeds – two tsp
- Natural peanut butter – two tsp
- Whole-wheat English muffin – one, toasted

Instructions:

- Place berries into the microwave and microwave it for a half minute.
- Stir it well and again microwave it for half-minute.
- Add in chia seeds. Scatter peanut butter over English muffins.
- Top with the chia-berry mixture.
- Serve!

Additional Tip:

- Garnish with berries.

Egg in a Hole Peppers with Avocado Salsa

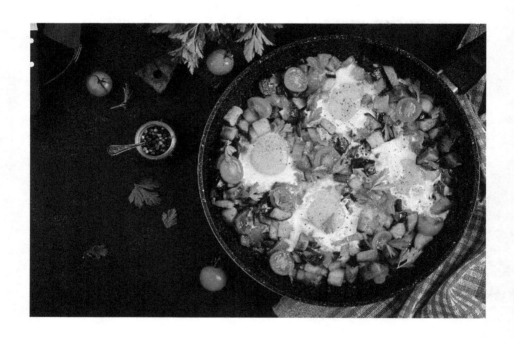

Preparation time: 5 minutes
Cooking time: 30 minutes
Serving: 4

Ingredients:

- Bell peppers – two, any color
- Avocado – one, diced
- Red onion – half cup, diced
- Jalapeño pepper – one, minced
- Fresh cilantro – half cup, chopped, for garnish
- Tomatoes – two, seeded and diced
- Juice of one lime
- Salt – ¾ tsp
- Olive oil – two tsp
- Eggs – eight
- Ground pepper – ¼ tsp

Instructions:

- Cut tops and bottom of the bell pepper and dice it.
- Remove the membrane and seeds of the bell pepper.
- Cut each bell pepper into rings.
- Mix the diced pepper with half tsp salt, lime juice, tomatoes, cilantro, jalapeno, onion, and avocado into the bowl.
- Add one tsp oil into the skillet and cook over medium flame.
- Then, add four bell pepper rings and break one egg into the center of each ring. Sprinkle with pepper and salt.

- Cook it for two to three minutes. Flip and cook for one minute more.
- Transfer it to the serving plate.

Additional Tip:

- Serve with avocado salsa.
- Sprinkle with cilantro leaves.

Egg and Vegetable Muffins

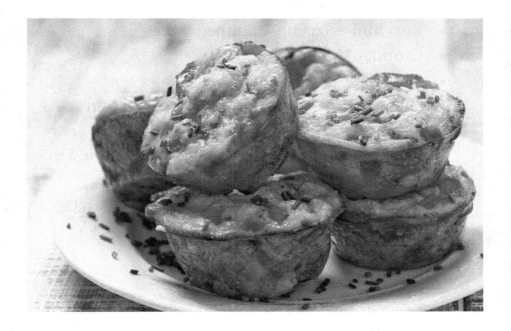

Preparation time: 5 minutes
Cooking time: 50 minutes
Serving: 6

Ingredients:

- Nonstick cooking spray – as needed
- Water – 2/3 cup
- Bulgur – 1/3 cup
- Zucchini – ¾ cup, chopped
- Onion – ¼ cup, chopped
- Olive oil – one tbsp
- One tomato – 1/3 cup, cored, seeded and chopped
- Reduced-fat feta cheese half cup, crumbled
- Eggs – two, beaten, frozen
- Snipped fresh oregano or rosemary – two tsp
- Ground black pepper – 1/8 tsp

Instructions:

- Preheat the oven to 350 degrees Fahrenheit.
- Coat two muffin cups with non-stick cooking spray. Keep it aside.
- Mix the bulgur and water into the saucepan and boil it. Lower the heat and simmer for twelve to fifteen minutes.
- Drain off any liquid. Then, add onion and zucchini in oil into the skillet and cook for five to ten minutes.
- Remove from the flame and then add in cheese, tomato, and bulgur.
- Add mixture into the muffin cups.

- Whisk the pepper, oregano, and eggs into the bowl. Add the vegetable mixture to muffin cups.
- Place into the oven and bake for fifteen to eighteen minutes.
- Let cool it for five minutes.
- Serve!

Additional Tip:

- Serve with butter.

Oatmeal Pancakes with Maple Fruit

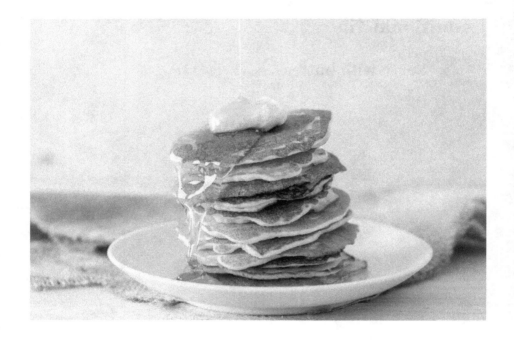

Preparation time: 10 minutes
Cooking time: 25 minutes
Serving: 8

Ingredients:

- Bananas – three, peeled and sliced
- Fresh blueberries – half cup
- Sugar-free maple-flavor syrup – ¼ cup
- Lemon juice – two tsp
- Ground cinnamon – ¼ tsp
- Flour – one cup
- Quick-cooking rolled oats – half cup
- Baking powder – 1 ½ tsp
- Baking soda – half tsp
- Salt – 1/8 tsp
- Low-fat buttermilk or sour milk – one cup
- One egg – beaten
- Canola oil – one tbsp
- Sugar-free maple-flavor syrup – one tbsp
- Vanilla – one tsp

Instructions:

- To prepare maple syrup: Add cinnamon, lemon juice, ¼ cup syrup, blueberries, and bananas into the bowl and stir well. Keep it aside.
- Add salt, baking soda, baking powder, oats, and flour into a bowl and stir well. Mix the vanilla, one tbsp syrup, egg, and buttermilk in the medium bowl using a fork.
- Add buttermilk mixture to the flour mixture and stir well. Let rest for ten minutes.

- For each pancake: Add two tbsp batter onto the griddle into a circle.
- Cook for one to two minutes over medium flame.

Additional Tip:

- Top with maple fruit.

Quark and Cucumber Toast

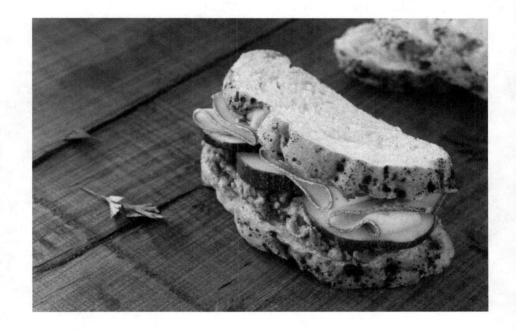

Preparation time: 5 minutes
Serving: 1

Ingredients:

- Whole-grain bread – one slice, toasted
- quark – two tbsp
- Cucumber – two tbsp, diced
- Cilantro leaves – one tbsp
- Pinch sea salt

Instructions:

- Add sea salt, cilantro, cucumber, and quark over the toast.
- Serve!

Additional Tip:

- Sprinkle with sea salt.

Breakfast Chocolate Chips Waffle

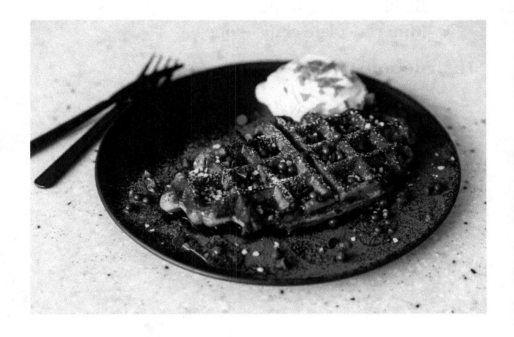

Cooking time: 5 minutes
Serving: 1

Ingredients:

- Whole-grain cinnamon waffle – one frozen
- Almond butter – one tbsp
- Banana – 1/4, sliced
- Mini chocolate chips – one tsp

Instructions:

- First, toast the waffle and scatter nut butter over it. Top with chocolate chips and sliced banana.
- Serve!

Additional Tip:

- Garnish with cookies.

Peanut Butter and Fig Crisp breads

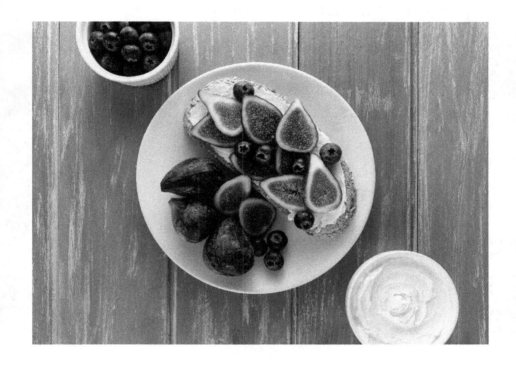

Preparation time: 5 minutes
Serving: 1

Ingredients:

- Crispbreads – two ryes
- Peanut butter – 2 tbsp
- Dried figs – four slices
- Pepitas – two tsp
- Coconut flakes – one tsp

Instructions:

- Top crispbread with half tsp coconut flakes, one tsp pepitas, half fig slices, and one tbsp peanut butter.
- Serve!

Additional Tip:

- Garnish with coconut flakes.

Cheddar and Zucchini Frittata

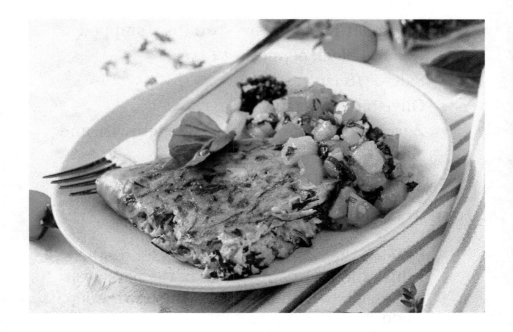

Preparation time: 5 minutes
Cooking time: 20 minutes
Serving: 4

Ingredients:

- Eggs – four
- Reduced-fat cheddar cheese – half cup, shredded
- Fresh flat-leaf parsley – two tbsp, snipped
- Ground black pepper – ¼ tsp
- Salt – 1/8 tsp
- Olive oil – two tsp
- Zucchini – 12 ounces, halved lengthwise and sliced
- Green onions – four, sliced

Instructions:

- Preheat the oven to 450 degrees Fahrenheit.
- Whisk the salt, pepper, half of the parsley leaves, cheese, and eggs into the bowl. Keep it aside.
- Add olive oil into the skillet and cook over medium-high flame.
- Then, add green onions and zucchini and cook for five to eight minutes until tender.
- Pour egg mixture over vegetables and then lower the heat to medium.
- Cook for five minutes until the egg mixture is set.
- Place the skillet into the oven and bake for five minutes.

Additional Tip:

- Sprinkle with two tbsp fresh parsley leaves.
- Slice into wedges and serve!

Orange Whole-Wheat Pancakes

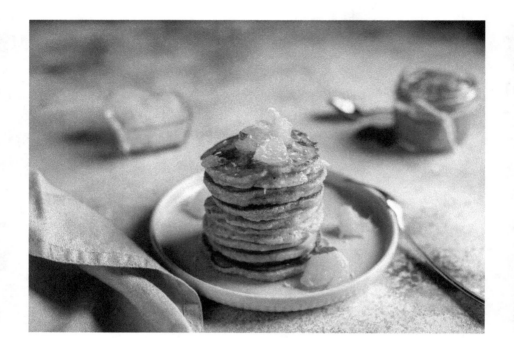

Preparation time: 5 minutes
Cooking time: 25 minutes
Serving: 6

Ingredients:

- White whole-wheat flour – 1 ½ cups
- Flaxmeal – three tbsp
- Baking powder – 1 ½ tsp
- Baking soda – half tsp
- Ground ginger – ¼ tsp
- Salt – 1/8 tsp
- Oranges – three
- Buttermilk – 1 ¼ cups
- Eggs – two
- Vanilla extract – one tsp
- Brown sugar – two tbsp
- Canola oil – two tbsp

Instructions:

- First, whisk the salt, ginger, baking soda, baking powder, flour, and flax meal into the bowl. Next, zest the one orange and juice it to get ¼ cup of juice.
- Slice the two oranges into segments and slice them into thirds and keep them aside.
- Whisk the zest, orange juice, oil, brown sugar, vanilla, eggs, and buttermilk into the bowl.
- Add the wet ingredients to the dry ingredients and mix it well.
- Let sit it for three to five minutes.
- Next, coat the pan with cooking spray and place it over medium-high flame. Add batter into the pan and cook for three to four minutes.

- Flip and cook for two to three minutes more.

Additional Tip:

Serve with orange segments.

Lunch recipes

Loaded Black Bean Nacho Soup

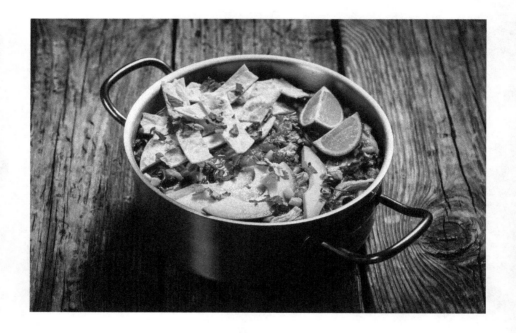

Cooking time: 10 minutes
Serving: 2

Ingredients:

- Low-sodium black bean soup – 18 ounces
- Smoked paprika – ¼ tsp
- Lime juice – half tsp
- Grape tomatoes – half cup, halved
- Cabbage or slaw mix – half cup, shredded
- Crumbled cotija cheese – two tbsp
- Avocado – half, diced
- Baked tortilla chips – 2 ounces

Instructions:

- First, add soup into the saucepan and then add paprika.
- Cook it and then add lime juice.
- Split the soup into two bowls.

Additional Tip:

- Top with avocado, cheese, slaw or cabbage, and tomatoes.
- Serve with tortilla chips.

Sautéed Spinach

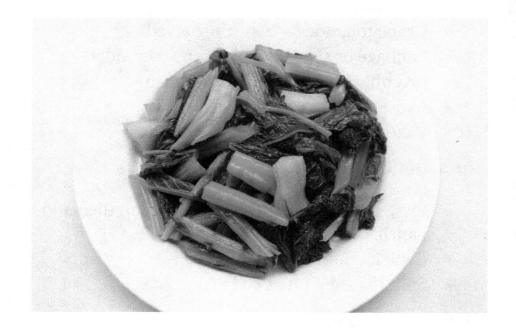

Cooking time: 10 minutes
Serving: 6

Ingredients:

- Extra-virgin olive oil – two tbsp
- Cloves garlic – four, thinly sliced
- Fresh spinach – 20 ounces
- Lemon juice – one tbsp
- Salt – ¼ tsp
- Red pepper – ¼ tsp, crushed

Instructions:

- Add oil into the Dutch oven and cook over medium flame.
- Add garlic and cook for one to two minutes.
- Then, add spinach and toss to combine.
- Cover with lid. Cook for three to five minutes.
- Remove from the flame. Then, add crushed red pepper, salt, and lemon juice.
- Toss to combine.
- Serve!

Additional Tip:

- Garnish with sesame seeds.

Spicy Chicken Fajitas

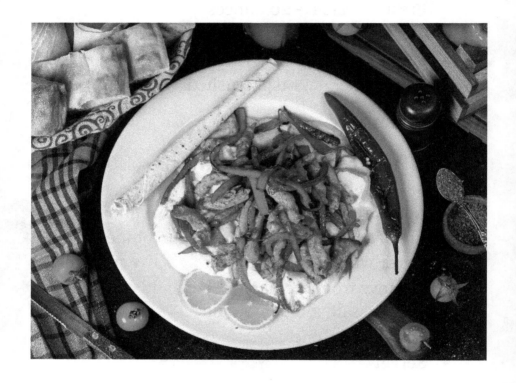

Preparation time: 20 minutes
Cooking time: 20 minutes
Serving: 4

Ingredients:

- Boneless, skinless chicken breasts – one pound
- Extra-virgin olive oil – two tbsp
- Chili powder – one tbsp
- Ground cumin – two tsp
- Garlic powder – one tsp
- Salt – ¾ tsp
- Red bell pepper – one, sliced
- Yellow bell pepper – one, sliced
- Red or yellow onion – two cups, sliced
- Lime juice – one tbsp
- Corn tortillas – eight, warmed
- Lime wedges, cilantro, sour cream, avocado and/or pico de gallo – for serving

Instructions:

- Preheat the oven to 400 degrees Fahrenheit.
- Let coat the rimmed baking sheet with cooking spray.
- Slice the chicken breasts in half horizontally and then cut them into strips.
- Mix the salt, garlic powder, cumin, chili powder, and oil into the bowl.
- Add chicken and coat with spice mixture. Add onion and bell peppers and stir well.
- Transfer the vegetables and chicken onto the baking sheet.
- Place into the oven and cook for fifteen minutes.

- Turn the broiler over high and broil it for five minutes more.
- Remove from the oven and then add lime juice.
- Serve in warm tortillas.

Additional Tip:

- Top with pico de gallo, avocado, sour cream, and cilantro.

Chickpea Curry

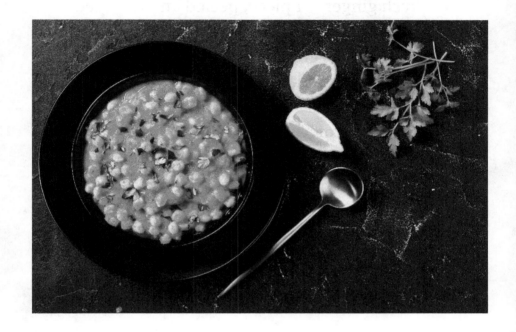

Cooking time: 15 minutes
Serving: 6

Ingredients:

- Serrano pepper – 1, cut into thirds
- Cloves garlic – four
- Fresh ginger – 1 piece, peeled and chopped
- Yellow onion – one, chopped
- Canola oil or grape-seed oil – six tbsp
- Ground coriander – two tsp
- Ground cumin – two tsp
- Ground turmeric – half tsp
- Tomatoes with their juice – 2 ¼ cups, diced
- Kosher salt – ¾ tsp
- Chickpeas – 15 ounce, rinsed
- Garam masala – two tsp
- Fresh cilantro – for garnish

Instructions:

- Add ginger, garlic, Serrano into the food processor and blend it.
- Add onion and pulse until chopped.
- Add oil into the saucepan and cook over medium-high flame.
- Add onion mixture and cook for three to five minutes until softened.
- Add turmeric, cumin, and coriander and cook for two minutes.
- Add tomatoes into the food processor and pulse until chopped.

- Add it to the pan with salt. Lower the heat and cook for four minutes.
- Add garam masala and chickpeas and lower the heat and cook for five minutes.

Additional Tip:

- Top with fresh cilantro.

Roast Chicken and Sweet Potatoes

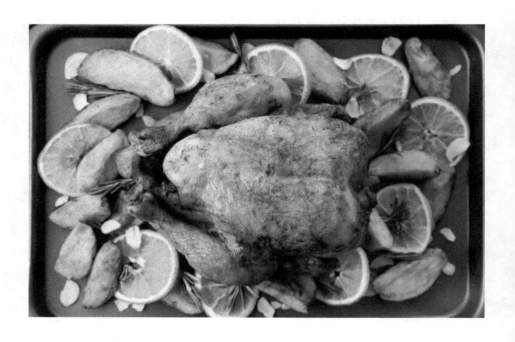

Cooking time: 45 minutes
Serving: 4

Ingredients:

- Dijon mustard – two tbsp
- Fresh thyme – two tbsp, chopped
- Extra-virgin olive oil – two tbsp
- Salt – half tsp
- Ground pepper – half tsp
- Bone-in chicken thighs – 1 ½ to 2 lb, skin removed
- Sweet potatoes – two, peeled and cut into 1-inch pieces
- Red onion – one, cut into 1-inch wedges

Instructions:

- Preheat the oven to 450 degrees Fahrenheit.
- Place the rimmed baking sheet into the oven.
- Mix the pepper, salt, one tbsp oil, thyme, and mustard into the bowl. Scatter the mixture on the chicken.
- Toss the onion and sweet potatoes with ¼ tsp pepper and salt and one tbsp oil. Remove the baking sheet from the oven and place vegetables on it. Add chicken over the vegetables.
- Place the pan back in the oven and cook for thirty to thirty-five minutes until tender.

Additional Tip:

- Garnish with fresh parsley leaves.

Delicious Ratatouille Dish

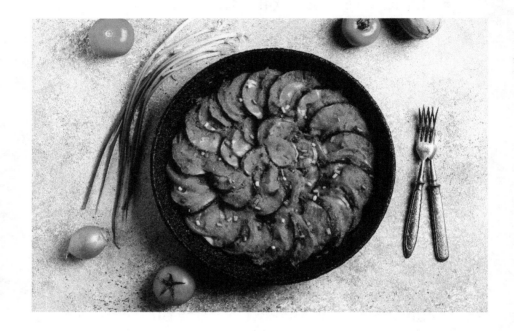

Cooking time: 1 hour and 25 minutes
Serving: 10

Ingredients:

- Extra-virgin olive oil – two tbsp
- Onions – two, chopped
- Red or yellow bell peppers – two, seeded and diced
- Cloves garlic – four, minced
- Fennel seeds – 1 ½ tsp, crushed
- Eggplant – one, diced
- Zucchini – two, diced
- Ripe tomatoes – six, chopped
- Fresh basil – ¼ cup, chopped
- Fresh thyme – two tbsp, chopped
- Salt and freshly ground pepper – as needed
- Fresh parsley – two tbsp, chopped

Instructions:

- Preheat the oven to 350 degrees Fahrenheit.
- Add one tbsp oil into the Dutch oven and cook over medium flame.
- Add bell peppers and onions and cook for eight to ten minutes.
- Add fennel seeds and garlic and cook for one minute more.
- Transfer the vegetables to the big bowl.
- Add one and a half tsp oil to the pot. Add eggplant and cook for seven to eight minutes until browned.
- Transfer it to the bowl with vegetables.

- Add remaining one and a half tsp oil to the pot. Then, add zucchini and cook for five minutes. Add reserved vegetables, thyme, basil, and tomatoes, and cover the pot with a lid. Place it into the oven and bake for thirty-five to forty-five minutes.

Additional Tip:

- Sprinkle with pepper and salt.
- Garnish with fresh parsley.

Roasted Baby Bok Choy

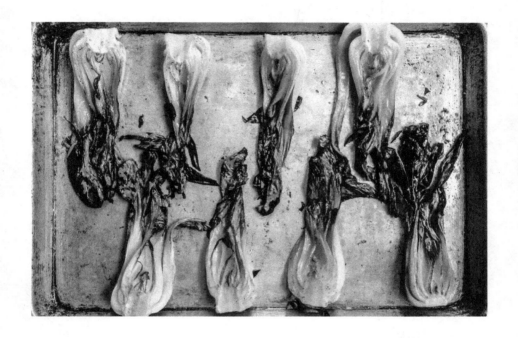

Cooking time: 15 minutes
Serving: 4

Ingredients:

- Baby bok choy – four heads, 1 1/4 pounds, trimmed, leaves separated
- Canola oil – four tsp
- Clove garlic – one, minced
- Kosher salt – ¼ tsp
- Freshly grated lemon zest – half tsp
- Lemon juice – one tbsp
- Fresh tarragon – 1 ½ tsp, chopped
- Mirin – one tsp
- Freshly ground pepper – as needed

Instructions:

- Preheat the oven to 450 degrees Fahrenheit.
- Toss the bok choy with salt, garlic, and oil into the roasting pan and cook for six minutes until tender.
- Whisk the pepper, mirin, tarragon, and lemon zest, and juice into the bowl.
- Add over roasted bok choy.
- Serve!

Additional Tip:

- Garnish with fresh basil leaves.

Roasted Zucchini and Pesto

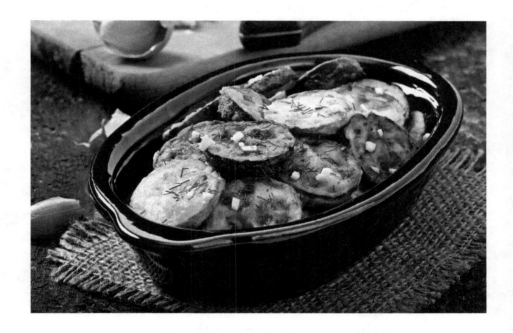

Cooking time: 25 minutes
Serving: 4

Ingredients:

- Zucchini – two pounds, trimmed and cut into 1-inch chunks
- Extra-virgin olive oil – one tbsp
- Prepared pesto – two tbsp
- Salt – as needed
- Freshly ground pepper – as needed

Instructions:

- First, preheat the oven to 500 degrees Fahrenheit.
- Toss zucchini with oil into the bowl. Scatter zucchini onto the baking sheet and cook for five to seven minutes.
- Turnover and cook for seven to nine minutes more.
- Place the zucchini back in the bowl.
- Add pepper, salt, and pesto and toss to combine.
- Serve!

Additional Tip:

- Garnish with fresh parsley leaves.

Paprika-Herb Rubbed Chicken

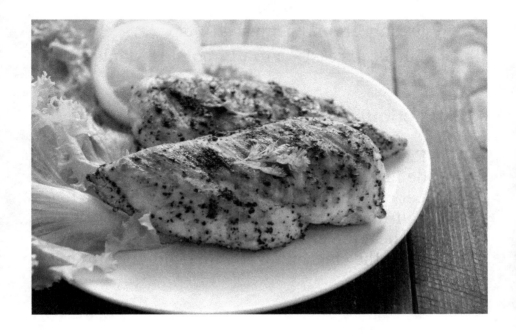

Cooking time: 25 minutes
Serving: 4

Ingredients:

- Herbes de Provence – one tbsp
- Paprika – two tsp
- Kosher salt – half tsp
- Freshly ground pepper – ¼ tsp
- Chicken breast – 1 to 1 ¼ pounds, skinless and boneless

Instructions:

- First, mix the pepper, salt, paprika, and herbes de Provence into the bowl.
- Let coat the chicken with seasoning for up to a half-hour before grilling.
- Preheat the grill over medium-high flame.
- Grill, the chicken for four to eight minutes per side.
- Serve!

Additional Tip:

- Sprinkle with pepper and salt.

Garlic-Sautéed Shrimp

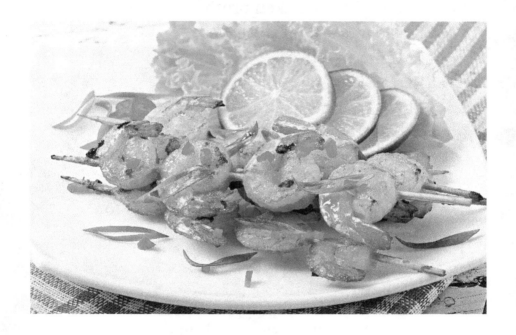

Cooking time: 40 minutes
Serving: 8

Ingredients:

- Raw shrimp – 24 unpeeled, with heads left on
- Dry white wine – ¾ cup
- Low-sodium chicken broth – ¾ cup
- Bay leaves – two bay leaves
- Butter – one tbsp
- Extra-virgin olive oil – one tbsp
- Clove garlic – one, thinly sliced
- Crushed red pepper – half tsp
- Kosher salt – ¼ tsp
- Lemon juice – two tsp, for garnish
- Fresh parsley leaves – one tbsp, plus for garnishing

Instructions:

- First, rinse the shrimp and pat it dry.
- Separate bodies from heads and peel all except tail and devein and keep it aside.
- Mix the shrimp shells and heads, bay leaves, broth, and wine into the skillet and boil it over medium-high flame.
- Lower the flame and cook for five minutes.
- Remove the lid and cook for three to five minutes more.
- Strain the stock into the medium bowl and remove the solids.
- Clean the pan. Add oil and butter into the pan and cook over medium-low flame.
- Add garlic and cook for one to two minutes.

- Add shrimp stock, salt, and crushed red pepper, elevate the heat to medium-high, and cook for three minutes.
- Place reserved shrimp into the pan and cook for one to two minutes per side.
- Then, add fresh parsley and lemon juice and toss to combine.
- Transfer the shrimp to the plate.

Additional Tip:

- Sprinkle with fresh parsley and lemon wedges.

Grilled Fish with Peperonata

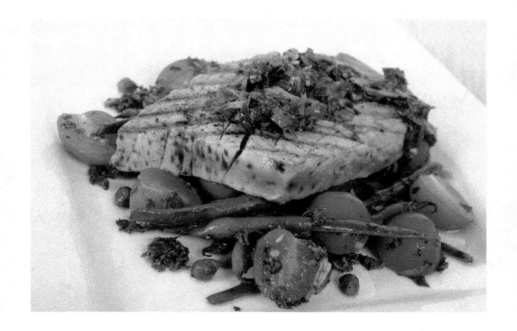

Cooking time: 45 minutes
Serving: 4

Ingredients:

- Extra-virgin olive oil – four tbsp
- Cloves garlic – three, thinly sliced
- Fennel seed – one tbsp
- pinch of crushed red pepper
- Red onion – one, thinly sliced
- Fresh oregano – one tsp, chopped
- Fresh thyme – one tsp, chopped
- Paprika – one tsp
- Bell peppers – eight cups, thinly sliced
- Capers – ¼ cup, rinsed
- Sherry vinegar – two tbsp
- Skinned banded rudderfish, amberjack, swordfish or mahi-mahi – 1 ½ pounds
- Kosher salt – half tsp
- Mixed tender fresh herbs, such as parsley, basil or mint – ¼ cup, chopped
- Fennel – ¼ cup, thinly sliced

Instructions:

- First, add two tbsp of oil into the pot and cook over medium-low flame.
- Add crushed red pepper, garlic, and fennel seed and cook for two to three minutes.
- Add onion and cook for five minutes. Add in paprika, thyme, and oregano and stir well.
- Add bell peppers and lower the heat to low, and cook for twenty minutes.

- Add vinegar and capers and cook for two minutes more.
- During this, preheat the grill over medium-high flame.
- Rub the fish with two tbsp oil and season with salt.
- Next, oil the grill rack. Place fish onto the grill and cook for six to ten minutes.
- Transfer the fish to the cutting board.
- Slice it into four parts.
- Place fish over pepperonata.

Additional Tip:

- Sprinkle with fennel and herbs.

Dinner recipes

Thai Peanut Shrimp Noodles

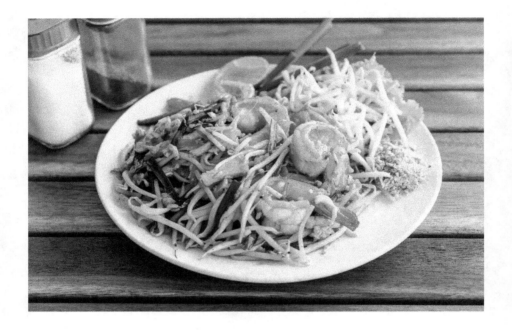

Cooking time: 5 minutes
Serving: 1

Ingredients:

- Cooked soba noodles – half cup, cooled
- Spiralized carrots – one cup
- Sugar snap peas – one cup, cut into thirds
- Shrimp – four, cooked, cooled
- Scallion – ¼ cup, sliced
- Peanut sauce – 1 ½ tbsp
- Fresh cilantro – two tbsp, chopped
- Unsalted peanuts – one tbsp, chopped

Instructions:

- Mix the scallion, shrimp, snap peas, carrots, and noodles into the bowl.
- Add peanut sauce and toss to coat.

Additional Tip:

- Season with peanuts and cilantro.

Crunchy Fish Amandine

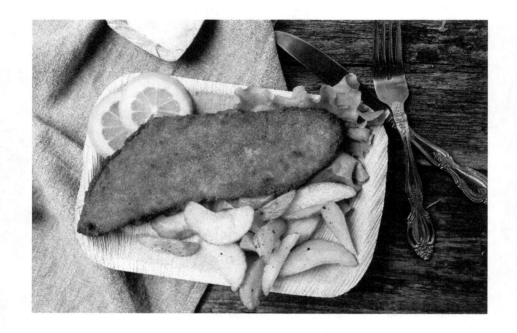

Cooking time: 15 minutes
Serving: 4

Ingredients:

- Fresh or frozen skinless tilapia, trout or halibut fillets – four ounces
- Buttermilk – ¼ cup
- Panko bread crumbs – half cup
- Fresh parsley – two tbsp, chopped
- Dry mustard – half tsp
- Salt – ¼ tsp
- Almonds – ¼ cup, sliced, chopped
- Grated Parmesan cheese – two tbsp
- Butter – one tbsp, melted
- Crushed red pepper – 1/8 tsp

Instructions:

- First, thaw fish if frozen.
- Preheat the oven to 450 degrees Fahrenheit.
- Let grease the baking pan and keep it aside.
- Wash the fish and pat it dry using paper towels.
- Add buttermilk to the dish. Mix the salt, dry mustard, fresh parsley, and breadcrumbs in another dish. Immerse the fish in buttermilk and then dip in the crumb mixture and coat it well. Place onto the baking pan.
- Sprinkle the fish with parmesan cheese and almonds.
- Drizzle with melted butter.

- Sprinkle with crushed red pepper. Place into the oven and bake for four to six minutes.
- Serve!

Additional Tip:

- Sprinkle with black pepper.

Turkey-Stuffed Bell Peppers

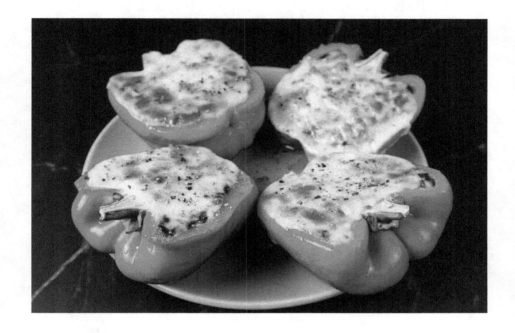

Preparation time: 30 minutes
Baking time: 20 minutes
Serving: 5

Ingredients:

- Green, red or yellow peppers – five
- Olive oil – two tsp
- Extra-lean ground turkey – 1-1/4 lbs
- Onion – one, chopped
- Garlic clove – one, minced
- Ground cumin – two tsp
- Italian seasoning – one tsp
- Salt – half tsp
- Pepper – half tsp
- Tomatoes – two, chopped
- Shredded cheddar cheese – 1-3/4 cups
- Soft bread crumbs – 1-1/2 cups
- Paprika – ¼ tsp

Instructions:

- Preheat the oven to 325 degrees Fahrenheit.
- Slice peppers in half and remove the seeds. Place onto the coated pan.
- Add oil into the skillet and cook over medium-high flame. Add seasoning, garlic, onion, and turkey and cook over medium-high flame for six to eight minutes. Let cool it.
- Add in breadcrumbs, tomatoes, and cheese.
- Next, fill the bell peppers with turkey mixture. Sprinkle with paprika. Place it into the oven and bake for twenty to twenty-five minutes.

- Serve and enjoy!

Additional Tip:

- Sprinkle with basil leaves.

Spicy Beef and Pepper Stir-Fry

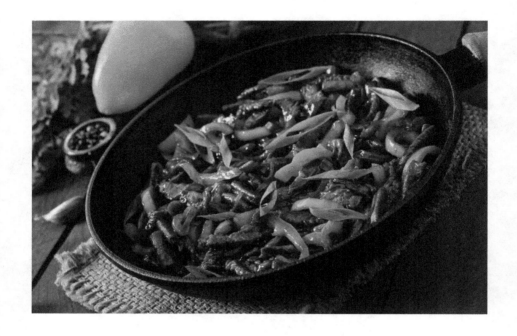

Cooking time: 20 minutes
Serving: 4

Ingredients:

- Beef top sirloin steak – one pound, cut into thin strips
- Fresh gingerroot – one tbsp, minced
- Garlic cloves – three, minced
- Pepper – ¼ tsp
- Salt – ¾ tsp
- Coconut milk – one cup
- Sugar – two tbsp
- Sriracha chili sauce – one tbsp
- Grated lime zest – half tsp
- Lime juice – two tbsp
- Canola oil – two tbsp
- Sweet red pepper – one, cut into thin strips
- Red onion – half, thinly sliced
- Jalapeno pepper – one, seeded and thinly sliced
- Fresh baby spinach – four cups
- Green onions – two, thinly sliced
- Fresh cilantro – two tbsp, chopped

Instructions:

- First, toss the half tsp salt, pepper, two garlic cloves, and ginger with beef into the bowl. Let stand for fifteen minutes.
- Whisk the remaining salt, lime juice, lime zest, chili sauce, sugar, and coconut milk into the bowl.

- Add one tbsp oil into the skillet and cook over medium-high flame.
- Add beef and cook for two to three minutes. Remove from the pan.
- Add remaining garlic, jalapeno, red onion, and red pepper in the oil and cook for two to three minutes. Add it to the coconut milk mixture.
- Add beef and spinach and cook until wilted.

Additional Tip:

- Sprinkle with cilantro and green onions.

Ginger Steak Fried Rice

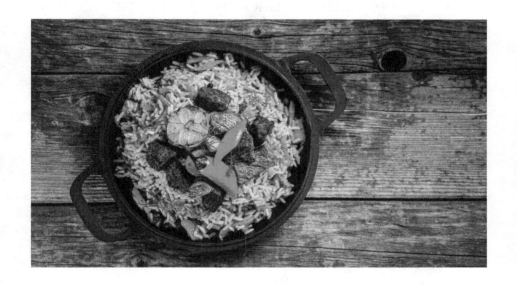

Preparation time: 5 minutes
Cooking time: 25 minutes
Serving: 4

Ingredients:

- Eggs – two, beaten
- Olive oil – two tsp
- Beef top sirloin steak – 3/4 pound, cut into thin strips
- Reduced-sodium soy sauce – four tbsp
- Broccoli coleslaw mix – 12 ounce
- Frozen peas – one cup
- Grated fresh gingerroot – two tbsp
- Garlic cloves – three, minced
- Cooked brown rice – two cups
- Green onions – four, sliced

Instructions:

- First, coat the skillet with cooking spray. Add egg and cook over medium flame.
- Remove from the pan and clean the skillet.
- Add oil in the same skillet and cook over medium-high flame.
- Add beef and cook for one to two minutes.
- Add in one tbsp soy sauce and remove from the pan.
- Add garlic, ginger, peas, and coleslaw mix to the pan and cook until tender.
- Add soy sauce and rice and toss to combine.
- Add in green onions, beef, and eggs and cook it well.

Additional Tip:

- Garnish with green onions.

Peppered Tuna Kabob

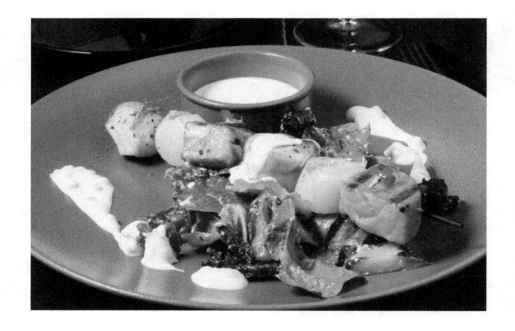

Preparation time: 5 minutes
Cooking time: 25 minutes
Serving: 4

Ingredients:

- Frozen corn – half cup, thawed
- Green onions – four, chopped
- Jalapeno pepper – one, seeded and chopped
- Fresh parsley – two tbsp, chopped
- Lime juice – two tbsp
- Tuna steaks – one pound, cut into 1-inch cubes
- Ground pepper – one tsp
- Sweet red peppers – two, cut into 2x1-inch pieces
- Mango – one, peeled and cut into 1-inch cubes

Instructions:

- **For the salsa:** Mix the corn, green onions, jalapeno pepper, parsley, and lime juice into the bowl. Keep it aside.
- Rub tuna with pepper—alternate thread the mango, tuna, and red pepper onto the soaked wooden skewers.
- Place skewers onto the greased grill rack and cook for ten to twelve minutes.
- Serve with salsa.

Additional Tip:

- Serve with mayonnaise.

and Rice Stuffed Cabbage Rolls

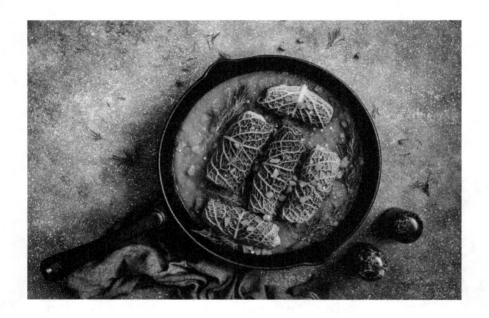

Preparation time: 20 minutes
Cooking time: 6 hours
Serving: 6

Ingredients:

- Cabbage leaves – 12
- Cooked brown rice – one cup
- Onion – ¼ cup, chopped
- Egg – one, beaten
- Fat-free milk – ¼ cup
- Salt – half tsp
- Pepper – ¼ tsp
- Lean ground beef – one pound

Sauce:

- Tomato sauce – 8 ounce
- Brown sugar – one tbsp
- Lemon juice – one tbsp
- Worcestershire sauce – one tsp

Instructions:

- Add cabbage in the boiled water and cook for three to five minutes until tender. Drain it.
- Trim the thick vein from each cabbage leaf.
- Mix the pepper, salt, milk, egg, onion, and rice into the bowl.
- Add beef and combine it well. Add ¼ cup of beef mixture onto each cabbage leaf. Fold over filling and fold it. Roll up.
- Place six rolls into the slow cooker. Mix the sauce ingredients into the bowl. Add half of the

sauce over cabbage rolls and top with sauce and remaining roll.
- Cook on low flame for six to eight hours.
- Serve!

Additional Tip:

- Squeeze lemon juice over it.

Chicken with Celery Root Puree

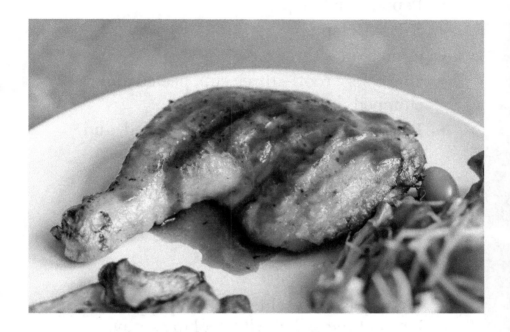

Preparation time: 30 minutes
Cooking time: 15 minutes
Serving: 4

Ingredients:

- Four boneless skinless chicken breast halves – 6-ounces each
- Pepper – half tsp
- Salt – ¼ tsp
- Canola oil – three tsp
- One celery root – three cup, peeled and chopped
- Butternut squash – two cups, peeled, and chopped
- Onion – one, chopped
- Garlic cloves – two, minced
- Unsweetened apple juice – 2/3 cup

Instructions:

- First, season the chicken with pepper and salt.
- Let coat the skillet with cooking spray.
- Add two tsp oil into the skillet and cook over medium flame.
- Cook until browned. Remove chicken from the pan.
- Take the same pan, add the remaining oil to it and cook over medium-high flame.
- Add onion, squash, and celery root and cook until tender.
- Add garlic and cook for one minute.
- Place chicken back in the pan. Add apple juice and boil it.

- Lower the heat and simmer for twelve to fifteen minutes.
- Remove chicken. Let cool the vegetable mixture.
- Add vegetable mixture to the food processor and place back to the pan and cook it.
- Serve with chicken and enjoy!

Additional Tip:

- Serve with sauce.

Ginger Salmon with Brown Rice

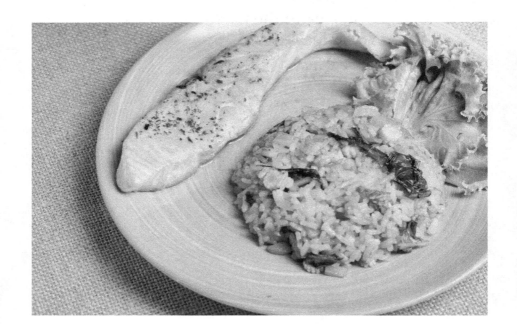

Preparation time: 25 minutes
Serving: 4

Ingredients:

- Four salmon fillets – six ounces each
- Reduced-fat sesame ginger salad dressing – five tbsp

Rice:

- 1/3 cup shredded carrot – 1/3 cup
- Green onions – four, chopped
- Instant brown rice – 1-1/2 cups
- Water – 1-1/2 cups
- Reduced-fat sesame ginger salad dressing – 1/3 cup

Instructions:

- Preheat the oven to 400 degrees Fahrenheit.
- Place fillets onto the baking sheet. Brush with three tbsp salad dressing. Place into the oven and bake for ten to twelve minutes.
- Brush with remaining salad dressing.
- During this, coat the saucepan with cooking spray and heat over medium flame.
- Add half of green onion and carrot and cook for two to three minutes.
- Add water and rice and boil it. Lower the flame and simmer for five minutes.
- Remove from the flame. Add in salad dressing and let leave it for five minutes.

- Serve with salmon.

Additional Tip:

- Top with green onions.

Turkey Stir-Fry

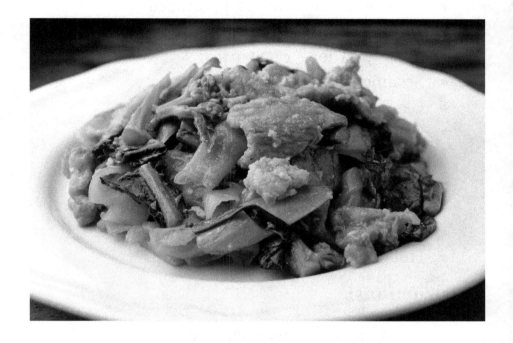

Preparation time: 5 minutes
Cooking time: 15 minutes
Serving: 4

Ingredients:

- Cornstarch – half tsp
- Reduced-sodium soy sauce – two tbsp
- Fresh cilantro – one tbsp, minced
- Honey – one tbsp
- Curry powder – one tsp
- Sesame or canola oil – one tsp
- Garlic clove – one, minced
- Crushed red pepper flakes – 1/8 tsp
- Canola oil – one tbsp
- Sweet red pepper – one, julienned
- Green onions – three, cut into 2-inch pieces
- Cubed cooked turkey breast – two cups
- Hot cooked brown rice – two cups

Instructions:

- Combine the cornstarch, soy sauce, cilantro, honey, curry powder, sesame or canola oil, garlic cloves, and pepper flakes.
- Add one tbsp canola oil into the skillet, cook over a medium-high flame, and cook for two minutes.
- Add green onion and cook for one to two minutes.
- Add in turkey and cook it well.

Additional Tip:

- Serve with rice.

Dessert recipes

Gingerbread Biscotti

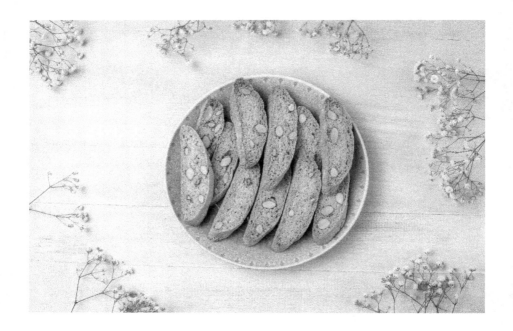

Preparation time: 25 minutes
Cooking time: 40 minutes
Servings: 48

Ingredients:

- Vegetable oil – 1/3 cup
- White sugar – one cup
- Eggs – three
- Molasses – ¼ cup
- All-purpose flour – 2 ¼ cups
- Whole wheat flour – one cup
- Baking powder – one tbsp
- Ground ginger – 1 ½ tbsp
- Ground cinnamon – ¾ tbsp
- Ground cloves – half tbsp
- Ground nutmeg – ¼ tsp

Instructions:

- Preheat the oven to 375 degrees Fahrenheit. Let grease the cookie sheet.
- Combine the molasses, eggs, sugar, and oil in a big bowl. Mix the nutmeg, cloves, cinnamon, ginger, baking powder, and flour in another bowl. Add it into the egg mixture and make stiff dough.
- Split the dough in half and roll the length of the cookie. Place this cookie onto the cookie sheet and bake it into the oven for twenty-five minutes.
- When done, remove it from the oven and keep it aside to cool.
- When cooled, slice it into diagonal slices.

- Place sliced biscotti onto the cookie sheet and bake it for five to seven minutes.
- Serve!

Additional Tip:

Garnish with nutmeg.

Rainbow Fruit Kebabs

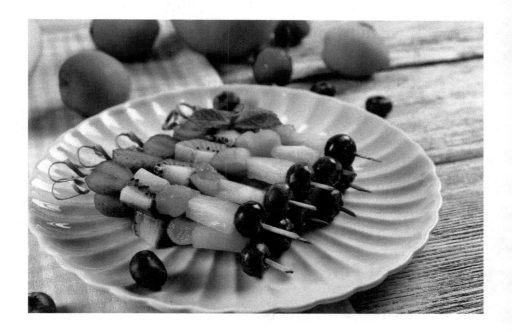

**Preparation time: 10 minutes
Serving: 2**

Ingredients:

- Strawberries – four
- Clementine – one, peeled
- Mango – half and cut into eight pieces
- Kiwifruit – one, peeled and quartered
- Blueberries – 1/3 cup
- Red seedless grapes – four

Instructions:

- Thread the grapes, blueberries, kiwi, mango, Clementine, and strawberries onto the four skewers.
- Serve and enjoy!

Additional Tip:

- Garnish with blueberries.

Sweet Mango Tiramisù

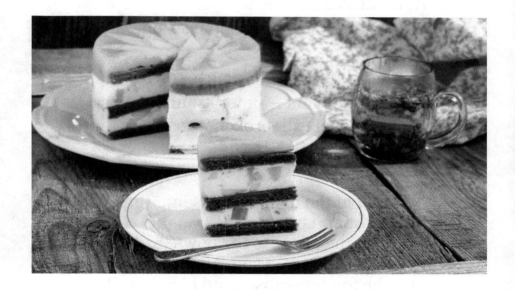

Preparation time: 30 minutes
Freezing time: 8 hours
Serving: 8

Ingredients:

- Two mangoes – two, cubed
- Light agave syrup – two tbsp
- Almond extract – ¼ tsp
- Frozen light whipped topping – one cup, thawed
- Nonfat vanilla Greek yogurt – one cup
- Crisp ladyfingers – 12 for example, Alessi Biscotti Savoiardi, broken into 1-inch pieces

Instructions:

- Add half of the mango cubes into the food processor and blend until smooth.
- Transfer the puree to the bowl. Add in almond extract and agave syrup. Add remaining mango into the food processor and blend until chopped. Keep it aside.
- Fold whipped topping into the yogurt in another bowl.
- Add half ladyfinger pieces onto the baking dish. Add half of the yogurt mixture and half of the mango puree over it.
- Top with chopped mango and again add remaining yogurt, puree, and ladyfingers.
- Cover the tiramisu with a plastic cover and place it into the fridge for eight to twenty-four hours.

Additional Tip:

- Garnish with mango.

Fluffy Key Lime Pie

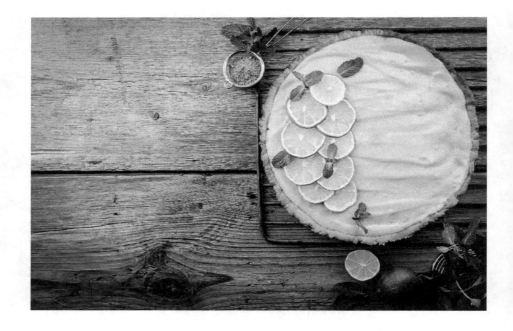

Preparation time: 20 minutes
Serving: 8

Ingredients:

- Boiling water - ¼ cup
- Sugar-free lime gelatin – 0.3 ounce
- Key lime yogurt – 12 ounce
- Frozen fat-free whipped topping – 8 ounce, thawed
- Reduced-fat graham cracker crust – one, 9 inches

Instructions:

- Add boiling water to the gelatin into the big bowl. Stir it for two minutes.
- Next, whisk in yogurt. Fold in the whipped topping and add it into the crust.
- Place it into the fridge for two hours with a lid.

Additional Tip:

- Garnish with mint leaves.

Mixed Berry Sundaes

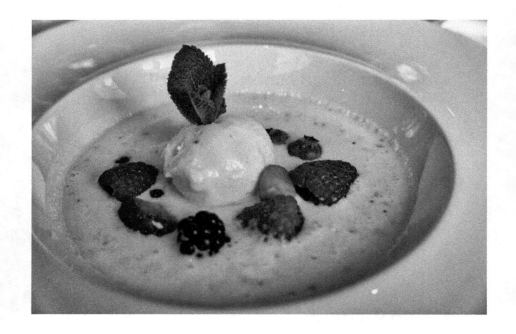

Preparation time: 10 minutes
Serving: 2

Ingredients:

- Fresh strawberries – ¼ cup, halved
- Fresh raspberries, blueberries and blackberries – ¼ cup each
- Honey – three tsp
- Fat-free plain Greek yogurt – half cup
- Pomegranate juice – two tbsp
- Walnuts – two tbsp, chopped, toasted

Instructions:

- Mix the one tsp honey and berries into the bowl. Add berries onto two dishes.
- Mix the remaining honey, pomegranate juice, and yogurt and add over the berries.

Additional Tip:

- Top with walnuts.

Best Banana Souffle

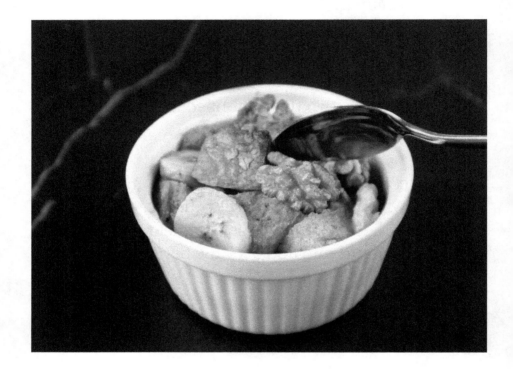

Preparation time: 30 minutes
Baking time: 25 minutes
Serving: 6

Ingredients:

- Eggs – four, separated
- Egg white – one
- Butter – two tbsp
- Ripe bananas – one cup, mashed
- Sugar – 1/3 cup
- Cornstarch – one tbsp
- Lemon juice – one tbsp
- Grated lemon zest – ¼ tsp

Instructions:

- Let stand the egg whites for a half hour.
- Coat the soufflé dish with cooking spray and keep it aside.
- Add butter into the saucepan and melt it.
- Add in cornstarch, sugar, and bananas and stir well. Let boil it for one to two minutes.
- Transfer it to the bowl. Add in lemon juice and lemon zest.
- Next, add a small amount of hot mixture into the egg yolks and place back in the bowl and stir well. Let cool it.
- Beat egg whites into the bowl using beaters.
- Add ¼ of egg whites into the banana mixture and stir it using a spatula.
- Fold in the remaining egg whites and transfer them to the dish.
- Place it into the oven and bake for twenty-five to thirty minutes.
- Serve!

Additional Tip:

- Garnish with sliced bananas.

Conclusion

I am very thankful to you because you choose my cookbook!
You will enjoy these recipes trust me! Keep following these simple rules in this cookbook to live a healthy and happy life!
Happy reading!